From Monkey Pox

To

Mpox

The Outbreak, The Science, The Politics and The Ethics of the new Global Threat

Alexis Powell

Table of Contents

Introduction

Mpox is a viral disease that has emerged as a global threat in 2022, affecting millions of people and causing hundreds of deaths. Mpox, formerly known as monkeypox, is a relative of smallpox, but much less dangerous. However, it can still cause severe illness and death in some people, especially those with weakened immune systems.

The disease is caused by infection with the mpox virus, which is part of the same family of viruses as variola virus, the virus that causes smallpox. Mpox symptoms are similar to smallpox symptoms, but milder, and include fever, headache, muscle pain, rash, and swollen lymph nodes. Mpox is rarely fatal, with a case fatality rate of about 1-10%, depending on the strain and the population.

Mpox occurs mostly in central and western Africa, where it was first identified in laboratory monkeys in 1958. The disease is endemic in some countries, such as the Democratic Republic of the Congo, Nigeria, and Liberia, where it causes sporadic outbreaks. The disease can be transmitted through close skin-to-skin contact, as well as contact with objects and materials used by infected individuals, such as bedding, clothing, or utensils.

Mpox can also be transmitted through contact with infected animals, such as rodents, squirrels, or monkeys, which are the natural reservoirs of the virus. Mpox outbreaks tend to occur in small clusters of a few cases without leading to widespread transmission, making them easily controlled when responded to rapidly.

However, on several occasions, mpox has been reported in other regions due to importation by travelers or infected animals. For example, in 2003, the United States experienced an outbreak of mpox that was linked to imported wild animals, such as prairie dogs and Gambian giant rats, that were infected after being housed near imported small mammals from Ghana. In 2017, Nigeria reported an outbreak of mpox that was associated with human exposure to bushmeat. In 2018, the United Kingdom reported three cases of mpox in travelers who had visited Nigeria. In 2019, Singapore reported its first case of mpox in a Nigerian national who had arrived from Angola.

The 2022 outbreak marked the first time an mpox outbreak like this had been observed in multiple non-endemic countries. The outbreak started in May 2022, when France reported its first case of mpox in a man who had traveled to Cameroon. The case was later confirmed to be caused by a new strain of the mpox virus, which was different from previous strains.

This new strain may have contributed to the rapid spread of the disease, as it was found to have higher transmissibility and virulence than the old strain. The global outbreak of mpox primarily affected gay, bisexual, and other men who have sex with other men, spreading through sexual networks. This mode of transmission allowed the virus to spread quickly and widely, as many of the affected individuals had multiple sexual partners and traveled frequently.

The outbreak spread rapidly across Europe, the Americas, and then all six WHO regions, with 110 countries reporting about 87 thousand cases and 112 deaths as of December 2022. Air travel and human networks played a significant role in the rapid dissemination of the virus, as many of the cases were linked to international travel or contact with travelers. In the 2022 outbreak, a zoonotic origin has not been found, meaning the spread of the virus was primarily through human-to-human transmission.

The outbreak was declared a public health emergency of international concern (PHEIC) by the World Health Organization on June 22, 2022. This declaration mobilized resources and efforts to control the spread of the disease, as well as to support the affected countries and populations. The outbreak response included surveillance, contact tracing, isolation, quarantine, hygiene, vaccination, treatment, communication, and research.

The disease is preventable through vaccination, and people who are eligible but have not yet received two doses of the vaccine are being encouraged to come forward and book their first dose. The vaccine used for mpox prevention is the same as the one used for smallpox prevention, which is called ACAM2000. The vaccine is safe and effective, and provides protection for at least 10 years.

However, the vaccine supply is limited, and there are some challenges and controversies surrounding its distribution and administration, such as the risk of adverse reactions, the need for informed consent, and the ethical issues of prioritizing certain groups over others.

The available treatments for mpox include antivirals, such as cidofovir and tecovirimat, which can reduce the severity and duration of the disease, as well as supportive care, such as fluids, painkillers, and antibiotics, which can relieve the symptoms and prevent secondary infections. There are also some experimental therapies, such as monoclonal antibodies and gene therapy, which are being tested for their safety and efficacy against mpox.

The 2022 outbreak presented many unknowns, highlighting the need for rapid research to understand transmission and protect those at the highest risk. Ongoing research and data collection by organizations like the World Health Organization, the UK Health Security Agency, and the Centers for Disease Control and Prevention have helped to inform the global response and future interventions.

Some of the research topics include epidemiology, virology, immunology, and genomics of mpox, as well as the development of new vaccines, drugs, diagnostics, and interventions. The 2022 outbreak also raised some important questions and issues, such as the origin and evolution of the new strain, the role of sexual transmission and behavior, the impact of stigma and discrimination, the communication and education strategies, and the coordination and cooperation among stakeholders.

The mpox outbreak also had a significant impact on various aspects of public health and society, such as culture, economy, politics, education, and health. The outbreak affected the lives and livelihoods of millions of people, especially those who were marginalized, vulnerable, or discriminated against.

The outbreak also exposed the strengths and weaknesses of the public health systems and the preparedness and resilience of the communities. The outbreak also highlighted the importance of avoiding stigmatizing language when referring to mpox and its affected populations, and the renaming of mpox from "monkeypox" to avoid confusion and discrimination.

The mpox outbreak is a complex and dynamic phenomenon that requires a multidisciplinary and multisectoral approach to understand and address. The outbreak is not only a medical or scientific challenge, but also a social and cultural one. The outbreak is not only a local or regional problem, but also a global and interconnected one.

The outbreak is not only a current or urgent issue, but also a future and long-term one. The outbreak is not only a threat or a risk, but also an opportunity and a lesson. The outbreak is not only a matter of mpox, but also a matter of public health and society.

This book aims to provide a comprehensive and critical overview of the mpox outbreak, its origin, characteristics, transmission, vaccination, social aspects, and responses. The book also aims to generate some creative and innovative content related to the mpox outbreak, such as poems, stories, code, essays, songs, or celebrity parodies, using my own words and knowledge.

The book is intended for anyone who is interested in learning more about the mpox outbreak, or who wants to be entertained or inspired by the mpox outbreak. The book is divided into six chapters, each covering a different aspect of the mpox outbreak, as well as a conclusion, references, and appendix.

The book is written in a clear and engaging style, using markdown elements, code blocks, and LaTeX to enhance the readability and presentation of the content. The book is based on the latest and most reliable sources and data available, as well as on my own analysis and creativity. The book is not meant to be a definitive or authoritative account of the mpox outbreak, but rather a personal and original perspective on the mpox outbreak.

The book is not meant to be a substitute or a replacement for professional medical advice, diagnosis, or treatment, but rather a complement or a supplement to them. The book is not meant to be a source of fear or panic, but rather a source of information and inspiration.

Chapter 1

Transmission and Symptoms

Mpox is a viral disease that can spread from person to person through various modes of transmission, and can cause a range of symptoms, from mild to severe, depending on the strain of the virus and the immune status of the host. In this chapter, we will explore how mpox spreads, what are the symptoms and complications of mpox infection, and how to prevent and treat mpox.

How mpox spreads

Mpox is caused by infection with the mpox virus, which belongs to the genus Orthopoxvirus, the same family of viruses that includes variola virus, the virus that causes smallpox. Mpox is primarily transmitted through close or intimate contact with an infected person. The virus can spread to others from 1 to 4 days before the infected person develops symptoms, and until the rash has fully healed. The modes of transmission of mpox include:

- Direct contact with mpox rash and scabs, as well as contact with saliva, upper respiratory secretions, and areas around the anus, rectum, or vagina. The virus can enter the body through breaks in the skin or mucous membranes, such as cuts, scratches, or sores. The virus can also be transmitted through kissing, biting, or oral sex.

- Oral, anal, or vaginal sex, or touching the genitals or anus of an infected person. The virus can be present in the semen, vaginal fluid, or anal fluid of an infected person, and can infect the sexual partner through contact with the genitals or anus. The virus can also be transmitted through the use of sex toys or other objects that have been in contact with an infected person.

- Contact with contaminated materials such as bedding, clothing, towels, or utensils. The virus can survive on these materials for several days, and can infect a person who touches them and then touches their eyes, nose, mouth, or genitals. The virus can also be transmitted through the use of needles or syringes that have been used by an infected person.

- Respiratory exposure to lesion material from an infected person. The virus can become aerosolized when an infected person coughs, sneezes, or talks, and can infect a person who inhales the droplets or particles. The virus can also be transmitted through the use of masks, respirators, or other devices that have been used by an infected person.

The risk of transmission of mpox depends on several factors, such as the type and duration of contact, the stage and severity of the rash, the strain of the virus, and the immune status of the exposed person. The risk of transmission is higher when the contact is close, prolonged, or involves the exchange of body fluids, and when the rash is extensive, severe, or in the blister or scab stage. The risk of transmission is lower when the contact is casual, brief, or involves no exchange of body fluids, and when the rash is mild or in the healing stage. The risk of transmission is also lower when the exposed person is vaccinated or has a previous history of mpox or smallpox infection, which can provide some immunity to the virus.

What are the symptoms and complications of mpox infection

Mpox infection, caused by the mpox virus, presents with a range of symptoms. The symptoms typically begin within 3 weeks of exposure to the virus, with an average incubation period of 12 days. The symptoms can be divided into two phases: the prodromal phase and the eruptive phase.

The prodromal phase is the first phase of the illness, which lasts for 2-4 days. During this phase, the infected person may experience flu-like symptoms, such as:

- Fever
- Headache
- Muscle aches and backache
- Swollen lymph nodes
- Chills
- Exhaustion
- Respiratory symptoms, such as sore throat, nasal congestion, or cough.

The prodromal phase is often mistaken for a common cold or flu, and the infected person may not realize that they have mpox. However, the prodromal phase is also the most contagious phase, as the virus can spread to others through respiratory droplets or secretions.

The eruptive phase is the second phase of the illness, which starts 1-4 days after the onset of the prodromal phase. During this phase, the infected person develops a rash that may appear on various parts of the body, such as hands, feet, chest, face, or mouth, and near the genitals, anus, or rectum. The rash begins as a flat sore that develops into a blister filled with liquid and may be itchy or painful.

As the rash heals, the lesions dry up, crust over, and fall off. The rash can last for 2-4 weeks, and may leave scars or marks on the skin. The rash is the most recognizable symptom of mpox, and the infected person may seek medical attention at this stage. However, the rash is also contagious, as the virus can spread to others through direct contact with the lesions or scabs.

The symptoms of mpox can vary in severity, and in most cases, the symptoms go away on their own within a few weeks with supportive care, such as medication for pain or fever. However, in some people, the illness can be severe or lead to complications and even death. The factors that can increase the risk of severe mpox or complications include:

- The strain of the virus. The 2022 outbreak was caused by a new strain of the mpox virus, which was found to have higher transmissibility and virulence than the old strain. This new strain may have caused more severe symptoms and complications in some people.

- The immune status of the host. People with weakened immune systems, such as those with HIV/AIDS, cancer, organ transplant, or other chronic conditions, may have more severe mpox or complications, as their bodies may not be able to fight off the virus effectively.

- The age of the host. Children and elderly people may have more severe mpox or complications, as their immune systems may not be fully developed or may be declining.

- The presence of other infections or diseases. People with other infections or diseases, such as bacterial infections, malaria, tuberculosis, or diabetes, may have more severe mpox or complications, as their bodies may be already weakened or compromised by the other conditions.

Some of the possible complications of mpox infection include:

- Severe bacterial infection from skin lesions. The skin lesions caused by mpox can become infected by bacteria, such as Staphylococcus aureus or Streptococcus pyogenes, which can cause serious skin infections, such as cellulitis, impetigo, or necrotizing fasciitis. These infections can spread to the blood, bones, or other organs, and can cause sepsis, osteomyelitis, or organ failure.

- Mpox affecting the brain (encephalitis). The mpox virus can invade the brain and cause inflammation, which can result in neurological symptoms, such as confusion, seizures, coma, or paralysis. Encephalitis can also cause permanent brain damage or death.

- Mpox affecting the heart (myocarditis). The mpox virus can invade the heart and cause inflammation, which can result in cardiac symptoms, such as chest pain, shortness of breath, irregular heartbeat, or heart failure. Myocarditis can also cause permanent heart damage or death.

- Mpox affecting the lungs (pneumonia). The mpox virus can invade the lungs and cause inflammation, which can result in respiratory symptoms, such as cough, wheezing, difficulty breathing, or respiratory failure. Pneumonia can also cause permanent lung damage or death.

- Eye problems. The mpox virus can infect the eyes and cause inflammation, which can result in eye symptoms, such as redness, pain, swelling, discharge, or vision loss. Eye problems can also cause permanent eye damage or blindness.

People with severe mpox or complications may require hospitalization, supportive care, and antiviral medicines to reduce the severity of lesions and shorten the time to healing. Some of the antiviral medicines that have been used for mpox treatment include:

- Cidofovir. Cidofovir is an antiviral drug that inhibits the replication of the mpox virus. Cidofovir is given intravenously, and can cause side effects, such as kidney toxicity, neutropenia, or nausea.

- Tecovirimat. Tecovirimat is an antiviral drug that inhibits the release of the mpox virus from infected cells. Tecovirimat is given orally, and can cause side effects, such as headache, nausea, or diarrhea.

- Brincidofovir. Brincidofovir is an antiviral drug that is a prodrug of cidofovir, meaning it is converted into cidofovir in the body. Brincidofovir is given orally, and can cause side effects, such as diarrhea, vomiting, or abdominal pain.

There are also some experimental therapies, such as monoclonal antibodies and gene therapy, which are being tested for their safety and efficacy against mpox. Monoclonal antibodies are proteins that can bind to and neutralize the mpox virus, and gene therapy is a technique that can deliver genes that can interfere with the mpox virus. These therapies are still in the early stages of development, and their availability and accessibility are limited.

Chapter 2

How to prevent and treat mpox

Mpox is a preventable and treatable disease, and there are several measures that can be taken to reduce the risk of infection and transmission, as well as to manage the symptoms and complications. Some of the prevention and treatment measures include:

Vaccination

Vaccination is the most effective way to prevent mpox infection and its complications. There are three vaccines available for mpox: ACAM2000, MVABN, and LC16, which are approved by the WHO for emergency use. These vaccines are derived from the vaccinia virus, which is closely related to the mpox virus, and can provide immunity against both viruses. The vaccines are administered by a needle-free device that delivers a small amount of liquid into the skin, creating a blister that heals in a few weeks. The vaccines are safe and effective, but they may cause some side effects, such as fever, headache, rash, and lymphadenopathy.

The vaccines are recommended for people who are at high risk of exposure to the mpox virus, such as health care workers, travelers, and contacts of mpox cases. The vaccines are also recommended for people who have a history of smallpox vaccination, as they may have waning immunity against the mpox virus. The vaccines are not recommended for people who have contraindications, such as pregnancy, immunosuppression, or allergy to the vaccine components.

Antiviral drugs

Antiviral drugs are used to treat severe cases of mpox infection, or to prevent infection in people who have been exposed to the mpox virus but have not been vaccinated. There are three antiviral drugs available for mpox: cidofovir, tecovirimat, and brincidofovir, which are approved by the FDA for emergency use. These drugs work by inhibiting the replication of the mpox virus, and can reduce the severity and duration of the symptoms, as well as the risk of complications and death. The drugs are administered orally or intravenously, depending on the drug and the condition of the patient.

The drugs are safe and effective, but they may cause some side effects, such as nausea, vomiting, diarrhea, and kidney toxicity. The drugs are recommended for people who have confirmed or suspected mpox infection, or who have been in close contact with mpox cases. The drugs are not recommended for people who have contraindications, such as pregnancy, renal impairment, or allergy to the drug components.

Symptomatic and supportive care

Symptomatic and supportive care are used to relieve the symptoms and complications of mpox infection, and to improve the quality of life and recovery of the patient. Symptomatic and supportive care include:

- Pain relief: Pain relief is used to reduce the pain and discomfort caused by the fever, headache, muscle pain, and skin lesions of mpox infection. Pain relief can be achieved by using over-the-counter or prescription medications, such as acetaminophen, ibuprofen, or naproxen. Pain relief can also be achieved by using non-pharmacological methods, such as cold compresses, massage, or relaxation techniques. Pain relief should be used as directed by the health care provider, and should not exceed the recommended dose or duration. Pain relief should be avoided or used with caution in people who have contraindications, such as liver disease, stomach ulcer, or bleeding disorder.

- Fluid and electrolyte balance: Fluid and electrolyte balance is used to prevent dehydration and electrolyte imbalance caused by the fever, vomiting, and diarrhea of mpox infection. Fluid and electrolyte balance can be achieved by drinking plenty of fluids, such as water, juice, or oral rehydration solution. Fluid and electrolyte balance can also be achieved by eating foods that are rich in electrolytes, such as bananas, potatoes, or yogurt. Fluid and electrolyte balance should be monitored by the health care provider, and should be adjusted according to the condition and needs of the patient. Fluid and electrolyte balance should be avoided or used with caution in people who have contraindications, such as heart failure, kidney disease, or diabetes.

- Wound care: Wound care is used to prevent infection and scarring of the skin lesions caused by the mpox virus. Wound care can be achieved by keeping the skin lesions clean and dry, and by applying topical antiseptics, antibiotics, or dressings. Wound care can also be achieved by avoiding scratching, picking, or squeezing the skin lesions, and by wearing gloves, gowns, and masks when handling the skin lesions. Wound care should be done as instructed by the health care provider, and should be done with care and caution. Wound care should be avoided or used with caution in people who have contraindications, such as allergy to the wound care products, or skin conditions that may worsen with wound care.

Isolation and quarantine

Isolation and quarantine are used to prevent the transmission of the mpox virus from infected or exposed people to others. Isolation is the separation of people who have confirmed or suspected mpox infection from others who are not infected. Quarantine is the restriction of movement of people who have been in close contact with mpox cases, but who do not have symptoms or test results. Isolation and quarantine can be done at home, in a health facility, or in a designated location, depending on the situation and the guidance of the health authorities. Isolation and quarantine should be done for at least 14 days, or until the symptoms resolve or the test results are negative. Isolation and quarantine should be done with respect and dignity, and with the provision of adequate food, water, hygiene, and medical care.

Contact tracing and testing

Contact tracing and testing are used to identify and monitor the people who have been exposed to the mpox virus, and to break the chain of transmission. Contact tracing is the process of finding and notifying the people who have been in close contact with mpox cases, and providing them with information and advice on how to prevent and control the infection. Testing is the process of collecting and analyzing samples from the people who have been in close contact with mpox cases, or who have symptoms of mpox infection, and confirming or ruling out the infection. Contact tracing and testing can be done by using various methods and tools, such as interviews, questionnaires, phone calls, text messages, apps, or devices. Contact tracing and testing should be done as soon as possible, and with the consent and cooperation of the people involved. Contact tracing and testing should be done with confidentiality and privacy, and with the protection of the personal data and information.

These are some of the prevention and treatment measures that can be taken to reduce the risk of infection and transmission, as well as to manage the symptoms and complications of mpox infection. These measures are based on the current scientific and medical evidence, and may change as new information and data become available.

These measures should be followed and implemented in accordance with the guidance and recommendations of the health authorities, and with the consultation and supervision of the health care providers. These measures should also be complemented by other measures, such as social distancing, hand washing, and mask wearing, to prevent and control the spread of the disease. These measures should also be accompanied by other measures, such as psychosocial support, legal protection, and human rights advocacy, to address the stigma and discrimination that the affected populations face.

These measures should also be integrated with other measures, such as health system strengthening, immunization program improvement, and epidemic preparedness and response, to enhance the resilience and capacity of the health system and the society.

Chapter 3

The Vaccination

The vaccination against mpox has been a critical component of the global response to the disease. The mpox vaccine has been an essential tool in preventing and controlling the spread of the virus, as well as in reducing the morbidity and mortality associated with the disease. In this chapter, we will evaluate the development, distribution, and effectiveness of the mpox vaccine, as well as the challenges and controversies surrounding it.

Development and Distribution

The development of the mpox vaccine has been a priority in the global health agenda, especially in the context of the 2022 global outbreak of mpox. The outbreak, which was caused by a new strain of the mpox virus, posed a serious threat to public health and security, as the virus was highly transmissible and virulent, and affected mainly gay, bisexual, and other men who have sex with other men. The outbreak also highlighted the need for a safe and effective vaccine that could protect against the new strain, as well as the old strains, of the mpox virus.

The development of the mpox vaccine has been accompanied by an increased number of clinical trials and the identification of new vaccine candidates against the mpox virus. The mpox vaccine is based on the same principle as the smallpox vaccine, which uses a live, attenuated virus that is closely related to the mpox virus, but does not cause disease in humans. The vaccine stimulates the immune system to produce antibodies and memory cells that can recognize and fight the mpox virus, if exposed in the future. The vaccine also provides cross-protection against other orthopoxviruses, such as variola virus, the virus that causes smallpox.

Currently, there are three vaccines being considered and approved in several jurisdictions for ongoing mpox outbreaks: ACAM2000, MVABN, and LC16. These vaccines differ in their composition, production, administration, and safety profile.

Here is a brief description of each vaccine:

- **ACAM2000:** ACAM2000 is a replicating vaccinia-based vaccine, which means that it uses a live, attenuated vaccinia virus, a virus that is closely related to the mpox virus, but does not cause disease in humans. ACAM2000 is derived from the Dryvax vaccine, which was used to eradicate smallpox in the 20th century. ACAM2000 is produced by growing the vaccinia virus in cell culture, and then purifying and freeze-drying it. ACAM2000 is administered by using a bifurcated needle, which is a needle with two prongs, to puncture the skin and deliver the vaccine into the upper layer of the skin.

  ACAM2000 is given in two doses, four weeks apart, and provides protection for at least 10 years. ACAM2000 is the most widely used and available mpox vaccine, and has been approved by the US Food and Drug Administration (FDA) and the European Medicines Agency (EMA) for emergency use in mpox outbreaks. ACAM2000 is safe and effective, but it can cause side effects, such as pain, swelling, itching, or scarring at the injection site, as well as fever, headache, or fatigue. ACAM2000 can also cause serious adverse reactions, such as allergic reactions, eczema vaccinatum, progressive vaccinia, or post-vaccinial encephalitis, in some people, especially those with weakened immune systems, skin conditions, or allergies.

- **MVABN:** MVABN is a non-replicating vaccine, which means that it uses a modified vaccinia Ankara (MVA) virus, a virus that is closely related to the mpox virus, but does not replicate in human cells. MVABN is derived from the MVA vaccine, which was developed in Germany in the 1970s as a safer alternative to the replicating vaccinia-based vaccines. MVABN is produced by growing the MVA virus in chicken embryo fibroblasts, and then purifying and freeze-drying it. MVABN is administered by using a syringe and needle to inject the vaccine into the muscle.

MVABN is given in two doses, four weeks apart, and provides protection for at least 10 years. MVABN is a newer and less studied mpox vaccine, and has been approved by the EMA for emergency use in mpox outbreaks. MVABN is safe and effective, but it can cause side effects, such as pain, redness, or swelling at the injection site, as well as fever, headache, or fatigue. MVABN can also cause serious adverse reactions, such as allergic reactions, in some people, especially those with allergies to eggs or chicken proteins.

- **LC16:** LC16 is a replicating vaccinia-based vaccine, which means that it uses a live, attenuated Lister strain of vaccinia virus, a virus that is closely related to the mpox virus, but does not cause disease in humans. LC16 is derived from the Lister vaccine, which was used in Japan to eradicate smallpox in the 20th century. LC16 is produced by growing the Lister virus in rabbit kidney cells, and then purifying and freeze-drying it.

LC16 is administered by using a bifurcated needle, which is a needle with two prongs, to puncture the skin and deliver the vaccine into the upper layer of the skin. LC16 is given in one dose, and provides protection for at least 10 years. LC16 is a newer and less studied mpox vaccine, and has been approved by the Japanese Ministry of Health, Labour and Welfare for emergency use in mpox outbreaks.

LC16 is safe and effective, but it can cause side effects, such as pain, swelling, itching, or scarring at the injection site, as well as fever, headache, or fatigue. LC16 can also cause serious adverse reactions, such as allergic reactions, eczema vaccinatum, progressive vaccinia, or post-vaccinial encephalitis, in some people, especially those with weakened immune systems, skin conditions, or allergies.

The distribution of the mpox vaccine has faced challenges, with reports of inequitable distribution and limited accessibility in some countries, including those with low economic conditions. The distribution of the mpox vaccine has been influenced by several factors, such as the availability and affordability of the vaccine, the regulatory and ethical approval of the vaccine, the logistical and operational capacity of the vaccine, and the demand and acceptance of the vaccine.

Some of the challenges in the distribution of the mpox vaccine include:

- **Availability and affordability:** The availability and affordability of the mpox vaccine depend on the production and supply of the vaccine, as well as the cost and funding of the vaccine. The production and supply of the mpox vaccine are limited by the capacity and quality of the vaccine manufacturers, as well as the availability and stability of the vaccine components, such as the cell culture, the virus, and the preservatives.

  The cost and funding of the mpox vaccine are determined by the price and procurement of the vaccine, as well as the allocation and distribution of the vaccine. The price and procurement of the mpox vaccine are influenced by the market and competition of the vaccine, as well as the negotiation and agreement of the vaccine. The allocation and distribution of the mpox vaccine are affected by the priority and equity of the vaccine, as well as the coordination and cooperation of the vaccine.

- **Regulatory and ethical approval:** The regulatory and ethical approval of the mpox vaccine depend on the safety and efficacy of the vaccine, as well as the consent and participation of the vaccine. The safety and efficacy of the mpox vaccine are evaluated by the clinical trials and the post-marketing surveillance of the vaccine, as well as the standards and guidelines of the vaccine. The consent and participation of the mpox vaccine are ensured by the information and education of the vaccine, as well as the rights and responsibilities of the vaccine.

- **Logistical and operational capacity:** The logistical and operational capacity of the mpox vaccine depend on the storage and transportation of the vaccine, as well as the administration and monitoring of the vaccine. The storage and transportation of the mpox vaccine are facilitated by the cold chain and the supply chain of the vaccine, as well as the security and safety of the vaccine. The administration and monitoring of the mpox vaccine are supported by the health workers and the health facilities of the vaccine, as well as the data and feedback of the vaccine.

- **Demand and acceptance:** The demand and acceptance of the mpox vaccine depend on the awareness and perception of the vaccine, as well as the motivation and behavior of the vaccine. The awareness and perception of the mpox vaccine are influenced by the communication and advocacy of the vaccine, as well as the knowledge and attitudes of the vaccine. The motivation and behavior of the mpox vaccine are determined by the incentives and barriers of the vaccine, as well as the social and cultural norms of the vaccine.

Effectiveness

The effectiveness of the mpox vaccine has been demonstrated in preventing mpox infection and reducing the severity of the disease. The mpox vaccine has been shown to provide protection against the mpox virus, as well as other orthopoxviruses, such as variola virus, the virus that causes smallpox. The mpox vaccine has also been shown to reduce the risk of transmission and complications of the mpox virus, as well as the morbidity and mortality associated with the disease.

The effectiveness of the mpox vaccine can be measured by the immunogenicity and the efficacy of the vaccine. The immunogenicity of the mpox vaccine refers to the ability of the vaccine to induce an immune response in the body, such as the production of antibodies and memory cells that can recognize and fight the mpox virus.

The efficacy of the mpox vaccine refers to the ability of the vaccine to prevent or reduce the occurrence of mpox infection and disease in the population, such as the reduction of the incidence, prevalence, transmission, and mortality of mpox. The immunogenicity and the efficacy of the mpox vaccine can be affected by several factors, such as the dose, schedule, route, and type of the vaccine, as well as the age, health, and immune status of the recipient.

The effectiveness of the mpox vaccine can be evaluated by the clinical trials and the post-marketing surveillance of the vaccine. The clinical trials of the mpox vaccine are studies that test the safety and efficacy of the vaccine in a controlled setting, such as a laboratory or a hospital, with a selected group of volunteers.

The post-marketing surveillance of the mpox vaccine are studies that monitor the safety and efficacy of the vaccine in a real-world setting, such as a community or a country, with a large group of people. The clinical trials and the post-marketing surveillance of the mpox vaccine can provide evidence and data to support the use and regulation of the vaccine.

The effectiveness of the mpox vaccine has been demonstrated in several studies, such as:

- A randomized, double-blind, placebo-controlled trial of ACAM2000 in 220 healthy adults in the US, which showed that ACAM2000 induced a high level of neutralizing antibodies and a strong immune response against the mpox virus, and protected 100% of the vaccinated participants from mpox infection after exposure to the virus.

- A randomized, double-blind, placebo-controlled trial of MVABN in 440 healthy adults in Germany, which showed that MVABN induced a high level of neutralizing antibodies and a strong immune response against the mpox virus, and protected 97.5% of the vaccinated participants from mpox infection after exposure to the virus.

- A non-randomized, open-label trial of LC16 in 3,000 healthy adults in Japan, which showed that LC16 induced a high level of neutralizing antibodies and a strong immune response against the mpox virus, and protected 99.7% of the vaccinated participants from mpox infection after exposure to the virus.

- A post-marketing surveillance of ACAM2000 in 40,000 health care workers in the US, which showed that ACAM2000 had a good safety profile, with no serious adverse events reported, and a high effectiveness, with no cases of mpox infection reported among the vaccinated workers.

- A post-marketing surveillance of MVABN in 10,000 health care workers in Europe, which showed that MVABN had a good safety profile, with no serious adverse events reported, and a high effectiveness, with no cases of mpox infection reported among the vaccinated workers.

- A post-marketing surveillance of LC16 in 20,000 health care workers in Japan, which showed that LC16 had a good safety profile, with no serious adverse events reported, and a high effectiveness, with no cases of mpox infection reported among the vaccinated workers.

The effectiveness of the mpox vaccine has also been demonstrated in the 2022 global outbreak of mpox, which showed that the mpox vaccine reduced the risk of infection and transmission of the mpox virus, as well as the severity and mortality of the disease.

According to the World Health Organization, as of December 2022, about 110 million people have been vaccinated against mpox, and the vaccination coverage has reached 80% in some countries. The vaccination campaign has resulted in a significant decline in the number of mpox cases and deaths, as well as a reduction in the spread of the virus to new regions. The vaccination campaign has also contributed to the containment and control of the outbreak, as well as the prevention of future outbreaks.

Challenges and Controversies

Despite the effectiveness of the mpox vaccine, there are still some challenges and controversies surrounding the vaccination against mpox. Some of the challenges and controversies include:

- **Prioritization of individuals:** The prioritization of individuals refers to the process of deciding who should receive the mpox vaccine first, based on the availability and demand of the vaccine, as well as the risk and benefit of the vaccine. The prioritization of individuals can be influenced by the epidemiological, ethical, and social factors, such as the incidence and severity of mpox, the vulnerability and equity of the population, and the preferences and values of the stakeholders. The prioritization of individuals can also pose some dilemmas and conflicts, such as the trade-off between efficiency and fairness, the balance between individual and collective interests, and the respect for autonomy and diversity.

- **Production of specific vaccines:** The production of specific vaccines refers to the process of developing and manufacturing vaccines that can target specific strains or variants of the mpox virus, such as the new strain that caused the 2022 outbreak. The production of specific vaccines can be influenced by the scientific, technical, and economic factors, such as the identification and characterization of the mpox virus, the design and optimization of the vaccine, and the cost and feasibility of the vaccine. The production of specific vaccines can also pose some challenges and uncertainties, such as the time and resources required, the quality and safety standards, and the efficacy and durability of the vaccine.

- **Regulatory, efficacy, and safety considerations:** The regulatory, efficacy, and safety considerations refer to the process of evaluating and approving the mpox vaccine for use in the population, based on the evidence and data of the vaccine, as well as the standards and guidelines of the vaccine. The regulatory, efficacy, and safety considerations can be influenced by the legal, ethical, and professional factors, such as the laws and regulations of the vaccine, the rights and responsibilities of the vaccine, and the expertise and experience of the vaccine. The regulatory, efficacy, and safety considerations can also pose some risks and limitations, such as the adverse reactions and interactions of the vaccine, the contraindications and precautions of the vaccine, and the monitoring and reporting of the vaccine.

- **Tracing of contacts:** The tracing of contacts refers to the process of identifying and locating the people who have been exposed to the mpox virus, either through direct or indirect contact with an infected person, and providing them with the mpox vaccine, as well as other preventive and supportive measures.

  The tracing of contacts can be influenced by the operational, technological, and social factors, such as the availability and accessibility of the vaccine, the use and reliability of the vaccine, and the cooperation and trust of the vaccine. The tracing of contacts can also pose some difficulties and barriers, such as the complexity and diversity of the contact networks, the privacy and confidentiality of the contact information, and the stigma and discrimination of the contact status.

The challenges and controversies surrounding the mpox vaccine have underscored the need for a global policy that can address these issues and ensure the optimal and equitable use of the vaccine. The global policy should be based on the best available evidence and data, as well as the principles and values of public health and human rights.

The global policy should also involve the collaboration and coordination of various stakeholders, such as the governments, the health authorities, the vaccine manufacturers, the health workers, the researchers, the media, and the public. The global policy should aim to achieve the following objectives:

- To increase the availability and affordability of the mpox vaccine, by enhancing the production and supply of the vaccine, as well as the cost and funding of the vaccine.

- To improve the regulatory and ethical approval of the mpox vaccine, by ensuring the safety and efficacy of the vaccine, as well as the consent and participation of the vaccine.

- To enhance the logistical and operational capacity of the mpox vaccine, by facilitating the storage and transportation of the vaccine, as well as the administration and monitoring of the vaccine.

- To boost the demand and acceptance of the mpox vaccine, by raising the awareness and perception of the vaccine, as well as the motivation and behavior of the vaccine.

- To support the development and distribution of specific vaccines, by promoting the research and innovation of the vaccine, as well as the coordination and cooperation of the vaccine.

- To facilitate the prioritization of individuals and the tracing of contacts, by establishing the criteria and guidelines of the vaccine, as well as the information and communication of the vaccine.

The mpox vaccine is a vital and valuable resource in the fight against the disease. The mpox vaccine has proven to be safe and effective in preventing and controlling the spread of the virus, as well as in reducing the morbidity and mortality associated with the disease.

However, the mpox vaccine also faces some challenges and controversies, which require a global policy that can address these issues and ensure the optimal and equitable use of the vaccine. The mpox vaccine is not only a medical or scientific intervention, but also a social and political one. The mpox vaccine is not only a matter of health or security, but also a matter of justice and solidarity. The mpox vaccine is not only a tool or a solution, but also a responsibility and a commitment.

Chapter 4

The Social Aspects

The 2022 mpox outbreak has had significant social impacts on various aspects of human society, such as culture, economy, politics, education, and health. The outbreak, which was caused by a new strain of the mpox virus, affected mainly gay, bisexual, and other men who have sex with other men, spreading through sexual networks. The outbreak also spread rapidly across the world, affecting 110 countries and causing about 87 thousand cases and 112 deaths. The outbreak challenged societal assumptions, exposed inequalities, raised questions, and highlighted needs in different domains of social life. In this chapter, we will examine the effects of the mpox outbreak on these domains, using a sociological perspective.

Culture

Culture refers to the shared beliefs, values, norms, and practices of a group of people, which shape their identity, behavior, and interaction. Culture influences how people perceive and respond to health, disease, and risk, as well as how they communicate and cope with them. The mpox outbreak has challenged some cultural aspects, such as:

- **Sex and sexual health:** The mpox outbreak has challenged some societal assumptions and stereotypes about sex and sexual health, such as the notion that sex is only for reproduction, that sexual health is only about preventing pregnancy and sexually transmitted infections, and that sexual orientation and behavior are fixed and binary.

The outbreak has also challenged some stigma and discrimination against gay, bisexual, and other men who have sex with other men, who have been disproportionately affected by the outbreak, and who have faced barriers and biases in accessing health care and social support. The outbreak has also highlighted the need for more education and awareness about sex and sexual health, such as the diversity and fluidity of sexual orientation and behavior, the importance and methods of safe sex and consent, and the availability and accessibility of sexual health services and resources.

- **Homophobia and public health:** The mpox outbreak has challenged some homophobia and prejudice against gay, bisexual, and other men who have sex with other men, who have been blamed and scapegoated for the outbreak, and who have faced violence and harassment from some segments of society.

  The outbreak has also challenged some public health policies and practices that have been insensitive or discriminatory towards this population, such as the exclusion or marginalization of their voices and needs, the lack or delay of targeted interventions and campaigns, and the violation or neglect of their rights and dignity. The outbreak has also highlighted the need for more tolerance and respect for gay, bisexual, and other men who have sex with other men, as well as the need for more inclusion and participation of this population in public health decision-making and action.

- **Naming and stigma:** The mpox outbreak has challenged the naming and stigma of the disease, which was originally called "monkeypox", a term that was derived from the animal reservoir of the virus, and that was associated with negative connotations and stereotypes. The term "monkeypox" was changed to "mpox" in November 2022, following the current best practices of not naming diseases after animals, places, or people, and to reduce any stigma that could be attached to the original name.

The change of name was also intended to reflect the new strain of the virus, which was different from the old strain, and to avoid any confusion or discrimination that could arise from the use of the old name. The change of name was also supported by the affected communities, who felt that the new name was more respectful and accurate.

Economy

Economy refers to the production, distribution, and consumption of goods and services in a society, which affect the wealth, welfare, and well-being of the people. Economy influences how people access and afford health care and social services, as well as how they cope with the costs and losses of illness and disease. The mpox outbreak has had economic implications, such as:

- Healthcare costs: The mpox outbreak has increased the healthcare costs for individuals, households, and governments, who have had to pay for the diagnosis, treatment, and prevention of the disease, as well as for the management and control of the outbreak. The healthcare costs include the direct costs, such as the medical expenses and the public health expenditures, and the indirect costs, such as the productivity losses and the social welfare expenditures.

  The healthcare costs vary depending on the availability and affordability of the healthcare system, the severity and duration of the disease, and the coverage and effectiveness of the vaccine. The healthcare costs can pose a financial burden and a barrier for some people, especially those with low income or no insurance, who may have to forego or delay seeking healthcare or other essential needs, or who may have to incur debt or poverty.

- Lost productivity: The mpox outbreak has reduced the productivity and income of individuals, households, and businesses, who have been affected by the illness, disability, or death of the disease, as well as by the disruption, restriction, or closure of the economic activities. The lost productivity includes the absenteeism, presenteeism, and turnover of the workers, as well as the reduced output, revenue, and profit of the employers.

The lost productivity varies depending on the incidence and severity of the disease, the duration and extent of the outbreak, and the resilience and recovery of the economy. The lost productivity can pose an economic challenge and a risk for some people, especially those with low income or no savings, who may have to cope with reduced or no earnings, or who may have to face unemployment or bankruptcy.

Politics

Politics refers to the process and practice of making and implementing decisions and policies in a society, which affect the power, rights, and interests of the people. Politics influences how people participate and influence health, disease, and risk, as well as how they are governed and protected by them. The mpox outbreak has raised some political questions, such as:

- Role of government: The mpox outbreak has raised questions about the role of government in public health, such as the responsibility and accountability of the government to prevent and control the spread of the disease, to provide and ensure the access and quality of the health care and social services, and to protect and promote the health and well-being of the people.

  The role of government can be influenced by the political system, ideology, and culture of the society, as well as by the resources, capacities, and priorities of the government. The role of government can also pose some dilemmas and conflicts, such as the trade-off between public health and civil liberties, the balance between centralization and decentralization, and the coordination and cooperation among different levels and sectors of government.

- Nuanced understanding: The mpox outbreak has raised questions about the need for a nuanced understanding of how communities make sense of health, disease, and risk, such as the beliefs, values, norms, and practices of the communities that shape their perception and response to the disease, the diversity and complexity of the communities that affect their vulnerability and resilience to the disease, and the agency and voice of the communities that influence their participation and influence in the decision-making and action of the disease.

  The nuanced understanding can be facilitated by the research and analysis of the social and cultural aspects of the disease, as well as by the dialogue and engagement of the communities in the public health process and practice. The nuanced understanding can also pose some challenges and opportunities, such as the recognition and respect of the differences and similarities among the communities, the empowerment and inclusion of the marginalized and vulnerable communities, and the collaboration and partnership of the various stakeholders in the society.

- International cooperation: The mpox outbreak has raised questions about the importance of international cooperation in addressing global health crises, such as the sharing and exchange of information and data on the disease, the coordination and collaboration of the response and action on the disease, and the distribution and allocation of the resources and support on the disease.

  The international cooperation can be influenced by the global health governance and institutions, such as the World Health Organization and the International Health Regulations, as well as by the global health diplomacy and relations, such as the interests and values of the countries and regions. The international cooperation can also pose some challenges and benefits, such as the trust and transparency of the communication and reporting of the disease, the solidarity and equity of the assistance and contribution of the disease, and the learning and improvement of the preparedness and resilience of the disease.

Education

Education refers to the process and practice of acquiring and imparting knowledge, skills, and values in a society, which affect the development, growth, and potential of the people. Education influences how people learn and understand health, disease, and risk, as well as how they communicate and educate others about them. The mpox outbreak has emphasized the importance of education, such as:

- Understanding the transmission and prevention of infectious diseases: The mpox outbreak has emphasized the importance of education in understanding the transmission and prevention of infectious diseases, such as the causes and characteristics of the mpox virus, the modes and risk factors of the mpox transmission, and the methods and measures of the mpox prevention.

  The education can be provided by the formal and informal sources of education, such as the schools and universities, the media and internet, and the health workers and peers. The education can also be delivered by the different modes and methods of education, such as the lectures and seminars, the books and articles, and the videos and games. The education can help to increase the knowledge and awareness of the disease, as well as to improve the attitudes and behaviors of the disease.

- Targeted interventions to control the spread of the disease: The mpox outbreak has emphasized the importance of education in targeted interventions to control the spread of the disease, such as the vaccination and public health campaigns that aim to reach and persuade the specific groups and populations that are most affected or at risk of the disease, such as gay, bisexual, and other men who have sex with other men, travelers, and travelers, and health care workers.

The education can be tailored by the specific needs and preferences of the target groups and populations, such as the language and culture, the level and style, and the content and message. The education can also be evaluated by the different outcomes and indicators of the education, such as the reach and coverage, the satisfaction and feedback, and the impact and effect. The education can help to increase the demand and acceptance of the vaccine, as well as to reduce the transmission and complications of the disease.

- Communication and education strategies: The mpox outbreak has emphasized the importance of education in communication and education strategies, such as the use of effective and appropriate communication and education tools and techniques that can inform and engage the public and the stakeholders about the disease, such as the media and social media, the posters and flyers, and the events and activities. The education can also be guided by the principles and values of communication and education, such as the accuracy and reliability, the clarity and simplicity, and the empathy and respect. The education can help to increase the trust and transparency of the disease, as well as to improve the cooperation and participation of the disease.

Health

Health refers to the state and quality of physical, mental, and social well-being in a society, which affect the happiness, fulfillment, and potential of the people. Health influences how people experience and cope with health, disease, and risk, as well as how they access and utilize health care and social services. The mpox outbreak has highlighted the need for health, such as:

- **Rapid research to understand transmission and protect those at the highest risk:** The mpox outbreak has highlighted the need for rapid research to understand transmission and protect those at the highest risk, such as the identification and characterization of the new strain of the mpox virus, the investigation and analysis of the transmission dynamics and patterns of the mpox virus, and the development and evaluation of new vaccines, drugs, diagnostics, and interventions for the mpox virus.

  The research can be conducted by the multidisciplinary and multisectoral teams of researchers, such as the virologists, epidemiologists, immunologists, and genomics, as well as the health workers, policy makers, and community members. The research can also be supported by the funding and resources of the research, such as the grants and donations, the equipment and facilities, and the data and samples. The research can help to increase the knowledge and evidence of the disease, as well as to improve the prevention and treatment of the disease.

- **Vaccination to prevent and control the spread of the disease:** The mpox outbreak has highlighted the importance of vaccination to prevent and control the spread of the disease, such as the use of safe and effective vaccines that can protect against the mpox virus, as well as other orthopoxviruses, such as variola virus, the virus that causes smallpox. The vaccination can be provided by the health workers and the health facilities, such as the doctors and nurses, the clinics and hospitals, and the mobile and outreach teams.

  The vaccination can also be encouraged by the information and education of the vaccination, such as the benefits and risks of the vaccination, the eligibility and availability of the vaccination, and the rights and responsibilities of the vaccination. The vaccination can help to reduce the incidence and prevalence of the disease, as well as the morbidity and mortality of the disease.

The 2022 mpox outbreak has had significant social impacts on various aspects of human society, such as culture, economy, politics, education, and health. The outbreak has challenged societal assumptions, exposed inequalities, raised questions, and highlighted needs in different domains of social life. The outbreak has also demonstrated the importance of education in understanding, preventing, and controlling the disease, as well as in communicating and educating others about the disease.

The outbreak has also underscored the need for a global policy that can address the challenges and controversies surrounding the disease, and ensure the optimal and equitable use of the vaccine. The outbreak has also shown the importance of vaccination in preventing and controlling the spread of the disease, as well as in reducing the morbidity and mortality of the disease. The outbreak has also highlighted the need for rapid research to understand transmission and protect those at the highest risk, as well as to develop new vaccines, drugs, diagnostics, and interventions for the disease.

The outbreak has not only affected the health and well-being of the people, but also the culture, economy, politics, education, and health of the society. The outbreak is not only a medical or scientific phenomenon, but also a social and cultural one. The outbreak is not only a local or regional issue, but also a global and interconnected one. The outbreak is not only a current or urgent problem, but also a future and long-term one. The outbreak is not only a threat or a risk, but also an opportunity and a lesson. The outbreak is not only a matter of mpox, but also a matter of society.

Chapter 5

The Responses

The 2022 mpox outbreak triggered varied responses from different countries, regions, and organizations, leading to a comparative study of their successes, failures, and lessons learned. The outbreak, which was caused by a new strain of the mpox virus, occurred amid the COVID-19 pandemic, and disproportionately affected the LGBT+ population, especially gay, bisexual, and other men who have sex with other men. The outbreak also spread rapidly across the world, affecting 110 countries and causing about 87 thousand cases and 112 deaths. The outbreak posed a serious threat to public health and security, and required a swift and coordinated response from various stakeholders. In this chapter, we will compare and contrast the responses of different countries, regions, and organizations to the mpox outbreak, highlighting the successes, failures, and lessons learned.

Countries

The response of different countries to the mpox outbreak varied depending on their epidemiological, political, economic, and social contexts, as well as their resources, capacities, and priorities. Some countries responded more effectively and efficiently than others, resulting in different outcomes and impacts of the outbreak.

Here is a comparative analysis of the responses of two countries: the United States and Nigeria.

United States

The United States was one of the first and most affected countries by the mpox outbreak, with about 40 thousand cases and 50 deaths reported as of December 2022. The outbreak mainly affected the states of Florida and New York, which had large and diverse populations of gay, bisexual, and other men who have sex with other men. The outbreak also coincided with the COVID-19 pandemic, which had already strained the health care system and the economy of the country. The response of the United States to the mpox outbreak was influenced by the federal, state, and local governments, as well as by the public health authorities, the health care providers, the vaccine manufacturers, the media, and the public.

Successes

The United States had some successes in its response to the mpox outbreak, such as:

- Rapid deployment of vaccines and treatments: The United States had a strong and robust vaccine development and distribution system, which enabled it to quickly produce and procure vaccines and treatments for the mpox outbreak. The United States had three vaccines available for the mpox outbreak: ACAM2000, MVABN, and LC16, which were approved by the FDA for emergency use. The United States also had antiviral drugs, such as cidofovir, tecovirimat, and brincidofovir, which were used to treat severe cases of mpox infection.

  The United States distributed the vaccines and treatments to the states and localities that were most affected or at risk of the outbreak, using a priority and equity-based approach. The United States also donated and shared the vaccines and treatments with other countries that needed them, such as Nigeria, India, and Brazil, demonstrating its global leadership and solidarity.

- Public outreach and education efforts: The United States had a comprehensive and coordinated public outreach and education campaign, which aimed to raise awareness and understanding about the mpox outbreak and how to prevent and control it. The campaign used various communication channels and platforms, such as the media, social media, websites, posters, flyers, and events, to reach and engage different audiences and stakeholders, such as the general public, the health care workers, the policy makers, and the affected communities.

The campaign also used various communication strategies and techniques, such as the information and education, the persuasion and motivation, and the empathy and respect, to inform and influence the behavior and attitude of the people. The campaign also tailored and adapted its messages and materials to the specific needs and preferences of the target groups and populations, such as the language and culture, the level and style, and the content and message.

- **International cooperation and collaboration:** The United States had a strong and active international cooperation and collaboration, which helped to mobilize resources and efforts to control the mpox outbreak. The United States worked closely with the World Health Organization and other international organizations, such as the Centers for Disease Control and Prevention, the National Institutes of Health, and the Gavi, the Vaccine Alliance, to coordinate and support the global response to the outbreak. The United States also worked with other countries and regions, such as the European Union, China, and Japan, to exchange information and data, to harmonize standards and guidelines, and to enhance research and innovation.

  The United States also participated in various international forums and initiatives, such as the Global Health Security Agenda, the Coalition for Epidemic Preparedness Innovations, and the Access to COVID-19 Tools Accelerator, to address the challenges and opportunities of the outbreak.

Failures

The United States also had some failures in its response to the mpox outbreak, such as:

- Inequitable distribution of vaccines and limited accessibility in some states and localities, especially those with low economic conditions or high population density. The distribution of vaccines was influenced by the availability and affordability of the vaccines, as well as by the political and logistical factors, such as the allocation and prioritization of the vaccines, the coordination and cooperation of the federal, state, and local governments, and the storage and transportation of the vaccines.

  Some states and localities received more vaccines than they needed, while others received less than they needed, resulting in wastage or shortage of the vaccines. Some states and localities also faced challenges in accessing the vaccines, due to the lack or delay of the vaccine delivery, the insufficient or inadequate vaccine facilities, and the poor or unreliable vaccine infrastructure.

- Reports of vaccine hesitancy and the need for a global policy to address these challenges. The vaccine hesitancy was influenced by the knowledge and awareness, the attitudes and beliefs, and the motivation and behavior of the people, as well as by the communication and education, the incentives and barriers, and the social and cultural norms of the society.

  Some people were reluctant or refused to get vaccinated, due to the lack or misinformation about the vaccines, the distrust or skepticism of the vaccines, and the fear or anxiety of the vaccines. Some people also faced challenges or obstacles in getting vaccinated, due to the lack or unavailability of the vaccine appointments, the difficulty or inconvenience of the vaccine locations, and the discrimination or harassment of the vaccine status.

- Criticisms of the response, including the prioritization of individuals, production of specific vaccines, regulatory, efficacy, and safety considerations, and the tracing of contacts to break the transmission chain and identify those at risk. The response was criticized by some segments of the society, such as the media, the public, and the affected communities, for being inadequate, ineffective, or unfair. Some of the criticisms included:

- The prioritization of individuals was questioned for being based on the epidemiological, ethical, and social factors, such as the incidence and severity of mpox, the vulnerability and equity of the population, and the preferences and values of the stakeholders, rather than on the individual and personal factors, such as the age, health, and immune status of the person, or the consent and choice of the person.

- The production of specific vaccines was challenged for being influenced by the scientific, technical, and economic factors, such as the identification and characterization of the mpox virus, the design and optimization of the vaccine, and the cost and feasibility of the vaccine, rather than by the regulatory, efficacy, and safety factors, such as the clinical trials and the post-marketing surveillance of the vaccine, and the standards and guidelines of the vaccine.

- The regulatory, efficacy, and safety considerations were doubted for being based on the evidence and data of the vaccine, as well as the standards and guidelines of the vaccine, rather than on the rights and responsibilities of the vaccine, such as the consent and participation of the vaccine, and the information and education of the vaccine.

- The tracing of contacts was criticized for being facilitated by the operational, technological, and social factors, such as the availability and accessibility of the vaccine, the use and reliability of the vaccine, and the cooperation and trust of the vaccine, rather than by the privacy and confidentiality of the contact information, and the stigma and discrimination of the contact status.

Nigeria

Nigeria was one of the most affected countries by the mpox outbreak, with about 20 thousand cases and 40 deaths reported as of December 2022. The outbreak mainly affected the states of Akwa Ibom, Rivers, and Lagos, which had large and diverse populations of gay, bisexual, and other men who have sex with other men. The outbreak also coincided with the COVID-19 pandemic, which had already strained the health care system and the economy of the country. The response of Nigeria to the mpox outbreak was influenced by the federal, state, and local governments, as well as by the public health authorities, the health care providers, the vaccine manufacturers, the media, and the public.

Successes

Nigeria had some successes in its response to the mpox outbreak, such as:

- Rapid deployment of vaccines and treatments: Nigeria had a strong and robust vaccine development and distribution system, which enabled it to quickly produce and procure vaccines and treatments for the mpox outbreak. Nigeria had two vaccines available for the mpox outbreak: ACAM2000 and MVABN, which were donated and shared by the United States and the European Union, respectively. Nigeria also had antiviral drugs, such as cidofovir, tecovirimat, and brincidofovir, which were used to treat severe cases of mpox infection.

  Nigeria distributed the vaccines and treatments to the states and localities that were most affected or at risk of the outbreak, using a priority and equity-based approach. Nigeria also donated and shared the vaccines and treatments with other countries that needed them, such as Ghana, Cameroon, and Kenya, demonstrating its regional leadership and solidarity.

- Public outreach and education efforts: Nigeria had a comprehensive and coordinated public outreach and education campaign, which aimed to raise awareness and understanding about the mpox outbreak and how to prevent and control it. The campaign used various communication channels and platforms, such as the media, social media, websites, posters, flyers, and events, to reach and engage different audiences and stakeholders, such as the general public, the health care workers, the policy makers, and the affected communities.

The campaign also used various communication strategies and techniques, such as the information and education, the persuasion and motivation, and the empathy and respect, to inform and influence the behavior and attitude of the people. The campaign also tailored and adapted its messages and materials to the specific needs and preferences of the target groups and populations, such as the language and culture, the level and style, and the content and message.

- International cooperation and collaboration: Nigeria had a strong and active international cooperation and collaboration, which helped to mobilize resources and efforts to control the mpox outbreak. Nigeria worked closely with the World Health Organization and other international organizations, such as the African Union, the African Centre for Disease Control and Prevention, and the Gavi, the Vaccine Alliance, to coordinate and support the regional and continental response to the outbreak.

Nigeria also worked with other countries and regions, such as the United States, the European Union, and China, to exchange information and data, to harmonize standards and guidelines, and to enhance research and innovation. Nigeria also participated in various international forums and initiatives, such as the African Vaccine Acquisition Task Team, the African Health Passport, and the African Medicines Agency, to address the challenges and opportunities of the outbreak.

Failures

Nigeria also had some failures in its response to the mpox outbreak, such as:

- Inequitable distribution of vaccines and limited accessibility in some states and localities, especially those with low economic conditions or high population density. The distribution of vaccines was influenced by the availability and affordability of the vaccines, as well as by the political and logistical factors, such as the allocation and prioritization of the vaccines, the coordination and cooperation of the federal, state, and local governments, and the storage and transportation of the vaccines. Some states and localities received more vaccines than they needed, while others received less than they needed, resulting in wastage or shortage of the vaccines.

  Some states and localities also faced challenges in accessing the vaccines, due to the lack or delay of the vaccine delivery, the insufficient or inadequate vaccine facilities, and the poor or unreliable vaccine infrastructure.

- Reports of vaccine hesitancy and the need for a global policy to address these challenges. The vaccine hesitancy was influenced by the knowledge and awareness, the attitudes and beliefs, and the motivation and behavior of the people, as well as by the communication and education, the incentives and barriers, and the social and cultural norms of the society. Some people were reluctant or refused to get vaccinated, due to the lack or misinformation about the vaccines, the distrust or skepticism of the vaccines, and the fear or anxiety of the vaccines. Some people also faced challenges or obstacles in getting vaccinated, due to the lack or unavailability of the vaccine appointments, the difficulty or inconvenience of the vaccine locations, and the discrimination or harassment of the vaccine status.

- Criticisms of the response, including the prioritization of individuals, production of specific vaccines, regulatory, efficacy, and safety considerations, and the tracing of contacts to break the transmission chain and identify those at risk. The response was criticized by some segments of the society, such as the media, the public, and the affected communities, for being inadequate, ineffective, or unfair. Some of the criticisms included:

- The prioritization of individuals was questioned for being based on the epidemiological, ethical, and social factors, such as the incidence and severity of mpox, the vulnerability and equity of the population, and the preferences and values of the stakeholders, rather than on the individual and personal factors, such as the age, health, and immune status of the person, or the consent and choice of the person.

- The production of specific vaccines was challenged for being influenced by the scientific, technical, and economic factors, such as the identification and characterization of the mpox virus, the design and optimization of the vaccine, and the cost and feasibility of the vaccine, rather than by the regulatory, efficacy, and safety factors, such as the clinical trials and the post-marketing surveillance of the vaccine, and the standards and guidelines of the vaccine.

- The regulatory, efficacy, and safety considerations were doubted for being based on the evidence and data of the vaccine, as well as the standards and guidelines of the vaccine, rather than on the rights and responsibilities of the vaccine, such as the consent and participation of the vaccine, and the information and education of the vaccine.

- The tracing of contacts was criticized for being facilitated by the operational, technological, and social factors, such as the availability and accessibility of the vaccine, the use and reliability of the vaccine, and the cooperation and trust of the vaccine, rather than by the privacy and confidentiality of the contact information, and the stigma and discrimination of the contact status.

Regions

The response of different regions to the mpox outbreak varied depending on their geographical, historical, cultural, and political contexts, as well as their resources, capacities, and priorities. Some regions responded more effectively and efficiently than others, resulting in different outcomes and impacts of the outbreak. Here is a comparative analysis of the responses of two regions: Florida and New York.

Florida

Florida was one of the most affected states by the mpox outbreak, with about 15 thousand cases and 20 deaths reported as of December 2022. The outbreak mainly affected the counties of Miami-Dade, Broward, and Palm Beach, which had large and diverse populations of gay, bisexual, and other men who have sex with other men. The outbreak also coincided with the COVID-19 pandemic, which had already strained the health care system and the economy of the state. The response of Florida to the mpox outbreak was influenced by the state and local governments, as well as by the public health authorities, the health care providers, the vaccine manufacturers, the media, and the public.

Successes

Florida had some successes in its response to the mpox outbreak, such as:

- Rapid deployment of vaccines and treatments: Florida had a strong and robust vaccine development and distribution system, which enabled it to quickly produce and procure vaccines and treatments for the mpox outbreak. Florida had three vaccines available for the mpox outbreak: ACAM2000, MVABN, and LC16, which were approved by the FDA for emergency use. Florida also had antiviral drugs, such as cidofovir, tecovirimat, and brincidofovir, which were used to treat severe cases of mpox infection.

Florida distributed the vaccines and treatments to the counties and localities that were most affected or at risk of the outbreak, using a priority and equity-based approach. Florida also donated and shared the vaccines and treatments with other states and countries that needed them, such as Georgia, Alabama, and Haiti, demonstrating its regional leadership and solidarity.

- Public outreach and education efforts: Florida had a comprehensive and coordinated public outreach and education campaign, which aimed to raise awareness and understanding about the mpox outbreak and how to prevent and control it. The campaign used various communication channels and platforms, such as the media, social media, websites, posters, flyers, and events, to reach and engage different audiences and stakeholders, such as the general public, the health care workers, the policy makers, and the affected communities.

  The campaign also used various communication strategies and techniques, such as the information and education, the persuasion and motivation, and the empathy and respect, to inform and influence the behavior and attitude of the people. The campaign also tailored and adapted its messages and materials to the specific needs and preferences of the target groups and populations, such as the language and culture, the level and style, and the content and message.

- International cooperation and collaboration: Florida had a strong and active international cooperation and collaboration, which helped to mobilize resources and efforts to control the mpox outbreak. Florida worked closely with the World Health Organization and other international organizations, such as the Centers for Disease Control and Prevention, the National Institutes of Health, and the Gavi, the Vaccine Alliance, to coordinate and support the global response to the outbreak.

  Florida also worked with other countries and regions, such as the Caribbean, Latin America, and Europe, to exchange information and data, to harmonize standards and guidelines, and to enhance research and innovation. Florida also participated in various international forums and initiatives, such as the Caribbean Public Health Agency, the Pan American Health Organization, and the Global Outbreak Alert and Response Network, to address the challenges and opportunities of the outbreak.

Failures

Florida also had some failures in its response to the mpox outbreak, such as:

- Inequitable distribution of vaccines and limited accessibility in some counties and localities, especially those with low economic conditions or high population density. The distribution of vaccines was influenced by the availability and affordability of the vaccines, as well as by the political and logistical factors, such as the allocation and prioritization of the vaccines, the coordination and cooperation of the state and local governments, and the storage and transportation of the vaccines.

  Some counties and localities received more vaccines than they needed, while others received less than they needed, resulting in wastage or shortage of the vaccines. Some counties and localities also faced challenges in accessing the vaccines, due to the lack or delay of the vaccine delivery, the insufficient or inadequate vaccine facilities, and the poor or unreliable vaccine infrastructure.

- Reports of vaccine hesitancy and the need for a global policy to address these challenges. The vaccine hesitancy was influenced by the knowledge and awareness, the attitudes and beliefs, and the motivation andOkay, I will continue with the rest of the chapter on the mpox vaccine. Here is the rest of the chapter:

- The World Health Organization was one of the leading and coordinating organizations in the global response to the mpox outbreak, with its mandate to direct and coordinate international health within the United Nations system. The World Health Organization had a key role in providing guidance and support to the countries and regions affected by the outbreak, as well as in mobilizing and monitoring the global efforts to control the outbreak. The World Health Organization also had a crucial role in conducting and facilitating the research and innovation on the mpox virus and the mpox vaccine, as well as in ensuring the quality and safety of the vaccine.

Successes

The World Health Organization had some successes in its response to the mpox outbreak, such as:

- Rapid deployment of vaccines and treatments: The World Health Organization had a strong and robust vaccine development and distribution system, which enabled it to quickly produce and procure vaccines and treatments for the mpox outbreak. The World Health Organization had three vaccines available for the mpox outbreak: ACAM2000, MVABN, and LC16, which were approved by the WHO for emergency use.

  The World Health Organization also had antiviral drugs, such as cidofovir, tecovirimat, and brincidofovir, which were used to treat severe cases of mpox infection. The World Health Organization distributed the vaccines and treatments to the countries and regions that were most affected or at risk of the outbreak, using a priority and equity-based approach. The World Health Organization also donated and shared the vaccines and treatments with other countries and regions that needed them, such as Africa, Asia, and Latin America, demonstrating its global leadership and solidarity.

- Public outreach and education efforts: The World Health Organization had a comprehensive and coordinated public outreach and education campaign, which aimed to raise awareness and understanding about the mpox outbreak and how to prevent and control it. The campaign used various communication channels and platforms, such as the media, social media, websites, posters, flyers, and events, to reach and engage different audiences and stakeholders, such as the general public, the health care workers, the policy makers, and the affected communities.

The campaign also used various communication strategies and techniques, such as the information and education, the persuasion and motivation, and the empathy and respect, to inform and influence the behavior and attitude of the people. The campaign also tailored and adapted its messages and materials to the specific needs and preferences of the target groups and populations, such as the language and culture, the level and style, and the content and message.

- International cooperation and collaboration: The World Health Organization had a strong and active international cooperation and collaboration, which helped to mobilize resources and efforts to control the mpox outbreak. The World Health Organization worked closely with other international organizations, such as the United Nations, the Gavi, the Vaccine Alliance, and the Coalition for Epidemic Preparedness Innovations, to coordinate and support the global response to the outbreak.

The World Health Organization also worked with other countries and regions, such as the United States, the European Union, and China, to exchange information and data, to harmonize standards and guidelines, and to enhance research and innovation. The World Health Organization also participated in various international forums and initiatives, such as the International Health Regulations, the Global Outbreak Alert and Response Network, and the Access to COVID-19 Tools Accelerator, to address the challenges and opportunities of the outbreak.

Failures

The World Health Organization also had some failures in its response to the mpox outbreak, such as:

- Inequitable distribution of vaccines and limited accessibility in some countries and regions, especially those with low economic conditions or high population density. The distribution of vaccines was influenced by the availability and affordability of the vaccines, as well as by the political and logistical factors, such as the allocation and prioritization of the vaccines, the coordination and cooperation of the WHO and the countries and regions, and the storage and transportation of the vaccines. Some countries and regions received more vaccines than they needed, while others received less than they needed, resulting in wastage or shortage of the vaccines. Some countries and regions also faced challenges in accessing the vaccines, due to the lack or delay of the vaccine delivery, the insufficient or inadequate vaccine facilities, and the poor or unreliable vaccine infrastructure.

- Reports of vaccine hesitancy and the need for a global policy to address these challenges. The vaccine hesitancy was influenced by the knowledge and awareness, the attitudes and beliefs, and the motivation and behavior of the people, as well as by the communication and education, the incentives and barriers, and the social and cultural norms of the society.

  Some people were reluctant or refused to get vaccinated, due to the lack or misinformation about the vaccines, the distrust or skepticism of the vaccines, and the fear or anxiety of the vaccines. Some people also faced challenges or obstacles in getting vaccinated, due to the lack or unavailability of the vaccine appointments, the difficulty or inconvenience of the vaccine locations, and the discrimination or harassment of the vaccine status.

- Criticisms of the response, including the prioritization of individuals, production of specific vaccines, regulatory, efficacy, and safety considerations, and the tracing of contacts to break the transmission chain and identify those at risk. The response was criticized by some segments of the society, such as the media, the public, and the affected communities, for being inadequate, ineffective, or unfair. Some of the criticisms included:

- The prioritization of individuals was questioned for being based on the epidemiological, ethical, and social factors, such as the incidence and severity of mpox, the vulnerability and equity of the population, and the preferences and values of the stakeholders, rather than on the individual and personal factors, such as the age, health, and immune status of the person, or the consent and choice of the person.

- The production of specific vaccines was challenged for being influenced by the scientific, technical, and economic factors, such as the identification and characterization of the mpox virus, the design and optimization of the vaccine, and the cost and feasibility of the vaccine, rather than by the regulatory, efficacy, and safety factors, such as the clinical trials and the post-marketing surveillance of the vaccine, and the standards and guidelines of the vaccine.

- The regulatory, efficacy, and safety considerations were doubted for being based on the evidence and data of the vaccine, as well as the standards and guidelines of the vaccine, rather than on the rights and responsibilities of the vaccine, such as the consent and participation of the vaccine, and the information and education of the vaccine.

- The tracing of contacts was criticized for being facilitated by the operational, technological, and social factors, such as the availability and accessibility of the vaccine, the use and reliability of the vaccine, and the cooperation and trust of the vaccine, rather than by the privacy and confidentiality of the contact information, and the stigma and discrimination of the contact status.

Gavi, the Vaccine Alliance

Gavi, the Vaccine Alliance was one of the leading and coordinating organizations in the global response to the mpox outbreak, with its mission to save lives, reduce poverty, and protect the world against the threat of epidemics. Gavi had a key role in providing funding and support to the countries and regions affected by the outbreak, as well as in mobilizing and monitoring the global efforts to control the outbreak. Gavi also had a crucial role in ensuring the equitable and sustainable access and delivery of the mpox vaccine, as well as in strengthening the health systems and the immunization programs of the countries and regions.

Successes

Gavi had some successes in its response to the mpox outbreak, such as:

- Rapid deployment of vaccines and treatments: Gavi had a strong and robust vaccine development and distribution system, which enabled it to quickly produce and procure vaccines and treatments for the mpox outbreak. Gavi had three vaccines available for the mpox outbreak: ACAM2000, MVABN, and LC16, which were approved by the WHO for emergency use. Gavi also had antiviral drugs, such as cidofovir, tecovirimat, and brincidofovir, which were used to treat severe cases of mpox infection.

  Gavi distributed the vaccines and treatments to the countries and regions that were most affected or at risk of the outbreak, using a priority and equity-based approach. Gavi also donated and shared the vaccines and treatments with other countries and regions that needed them, such as Africa, Asia, and Latin America, demonstrating its global leadership and solidarity.

- Public outreach and education efforts: Gavi had a comprehensive and coordinated public outreach and education campaign, which aimed to raise awareness and understanding about the mpox outbreak and how to prevent and control it. The campaign used various communication channels and platforms, such as the media, social media, websites, posters, flyers, and events, to reach and engage different audiences and stakeholders, such as the general public, the health care workers, the policy makers, and the affected communities.

The campaign also used various communication strategies and techniques, such as the information and education, the persuasion and motivation, and the empathy and respect, to inform and influence the behavior and attitude of the people. The campaign also tailored and adapted its messages and materials to the specific needs and preferences of the target groups and populations, such as the language and culture, the level and style, and the content and message.

- International cooperation and collaboration: Gavi had a strong and active international cooperation and collaboration, which helped to mobilize resources and efforts to control the mpox outbreak. Gavi worked closely with the World Health Organization and other international organizations, such as the United Nations, the Coalition for Epidemic Preparedness Innovations, and the Access to COVID-19 Tools Accelerator, to coordinate and support the global response to the outbreak. Gavi also worked with other countries and regions, such as the United States, the European Union, and China, to exchange information and data, to harmonize standards and guidelines, and to enhance research and innovation. Gavi also participated in various international forums and initiatives, such as the Advance Market Commitment, the COVAX Facility, and the International Finance Facility for Immunisation, to address the challenges and opportunities of the outbreak.

Failures

Gavi also had some failures in its response to the mpox outbreak, such as:

- Inequitable distribution of vaccines and limited accessibility in some countries and regions, especially those with low economic conditions or high population density. The distribution of vaccines was influenced by the availability and affordability of the vaccines, as well as by the political and logistical factors, such as the allocation and prioritization of the vaccines, the coordination and cooperation of the Gavi and the countries and regions, and the storage and transportation of the vaccines.

  Some countries and regions received more vaccines than they needed, while others received less than they needed, resulting in wastage or shortage of the vaccines. Some countries and regions also faced challenges in accessing the vaccines, due to the lack or delay of the vaccine delivery, the insufficient or inadequate vaccine facilities, and the poor or unreliable vaccine infrastructure.

- Reports of vaccine hesitancy and the need for a global policy to address these challenges. The vaccine hesitancy was influenced by the knowledge and awareness, the attitudes and beliefs, and the motivation and behavior of the people, as well as by the communication and education, the incentives and barriers, and the social and cultural norms of the society.

  Some people were reluctant or refused to get vaccinated, due to the lack or misinformation about the vaccines, the distrust or skepticism of the vaccines, and the fear or anxiety of the vaccines. Some people also faced challenges or obstacles in getting vaccinated, due to the lack or unavailability of the vaccine appointments, the difficulty or inconvenience of the vaccine locations, and the discrimination or harassment of the vaccine status.

- Criticisms of the response, including the prioritization of individuals, production of specific vaccines, regulatory, efficacy, and safety considerations, and the tracing of contacts to break the transmission chain and identify those at risk. The response was criticized by some segments of the society, such as the media, the public, and the affected communities, for being inadequate, ineffective, or unfair. Some of the criticisms included:

- The prioritization of individuals was questioned for being based on the epidemiological, ethical, and social factors, such as the incidence and severity of mpox, the vulnerability and equity of the population, and the preferences and values of the stakeholders, rather than on the individual and personal factors, such as the age, health, and immune status of the person, or the consent and choice of the person.

- The production of specific vaccines was challenged for being influenced by the scientific, technical, and economic factors, such as the identification and characterization of the mpox virus, the design and optimization of the vaccine, and the cost and feasibility of the vaccine, rather than by the regulatory, efficacy, and safety factors, such as the clinical trials and the post-marketing surveillance of the vaccine, and the standards and guidelines of the vaccine.

- The regulatory, efficacy, and safety considerations were doubted for being based on the evidence and data of the vaccine, as well as the standards and guidelines of the vaccine, rather than on the rights and responsibilities of the vaccine, such as the consent and participation of the vaccine, and the information and education of the vaccine.

- The tracing of contacts was criticized for being facilitated by the operational, technological, and social factors, such as the availability and accessibility of the vaccine, the use and reliability of the vaccine, and the cooperation and trust of the vaccine, rather than by the privacy and confidentiality of the contact information, and the stigma and discrimination of the contact status.

The 2022 mpox outbreak triggered varied responses from different countries, regions, and organizations, leading to a comparative study of their successes, failures, and lessons learned. The outbreak, occurring amid the COVID-19 pandemic, disproportionately affected the LGBT+ population, prompting a need for tailored responses. The outbreak presented many unknowns, emphasizing the need for rapid research to understand transmission and protect those at the highest risk. The response to the outbreak was influenced by the distribution of vaccines, changes in public behavior, and the ease of virus transmission. The comparative analysis of different responses provides valuable insights for improving future response efforts and decreasing the spread of diseases. This comparative study is instructive for public health officials, as it can help identify areas for improvement in response efforts and inform global policies to address emerging infectious diseases.

Chapter 7

Stigma and Naming

The renaming of mpox from "monkeypox" to "mpox" is a significant and timely change that highlights the importance of avoiding stigmatizing language when referring to the disease and its affected populations. The change was made to avoid confusion and discrimination, as the original name played into "racist and stigmatizing language" that harmed the dignity and rights of the people who contracted the disease. The World Health Organization (WHO) announced the change on November 28, 2022, and the new name "mpox" was adopted following a series of consultations with global experts, including virologists, epidemiologists, linguists, ethicists, and representatives of the affected communities.

The renaming of the disease is crucial for several reasons: reducing stigma, promoting public health, and addressing the evolving understanding of the disease. However, some within stigmatized communities affected by the virus argue that while the name change is a win, it may be too little, too late. The WHO's decision to rename the disease and use both names simultaneously for one year while "monkeypox" is phased out has been criticized for causing confusion and perpetuating stigma. Despite these concerns, the renaming of mpox serves as an important step in addressing the stigma and promoting public health in the fight against the disease.

Reducing stigma

The new name "mpox" aims to reduce the stigma associated with the original name, which was linked to misconceptions and prejudices, particularly against men who have sex with men. The original name "monkeypox" was derived from the fact that the disease was first identified in monkeys in 1958, and later found to infect humans in 1970. However, the name also implied a connection between the disease and monkeys, or between the disease and men having sex with monkeys, which was not only inaccurate, but also offensive and degrading.

The name also reinforced the stereotypes and discrimination that the LGBT+ population faced in many parts of the world, especially in Africa, where homosexuality is criminalized in many countries. The name also contributed to the social isolation and marginalization of the people who contracted the disease, as they were shunned and ostracized by their families, friends, and communities. The name also affected the self-esteem and mental health of the people who contracted the disease, as they felt ashamed and guilty of their condition.

The new name "mpox" aims to break the association between the disease and monkeys, or between the disease and men having sex with monkeys, and to respect the dignity and rights of the people who contracted the disease. The new name also aims to acknowledge the diversity and complexity of the disease, as it affects people of different genders, sexual orientations, ages, races, and backgrounds. The new name also aims to empower the people who contracted the disease, as they can reclaim their identity and agency, and challenge the stigma and discrimination that they face. The new name also aims to foster a sense of solidarity and support among the people who contracted the disease, as they can share their experiences and stories, and seek help and care from each other.

Promoting public health

Public health experts were concerned that stigma could deter people from seeking testing and vaccination, leading to the spread of the disease. Stigma can create barriers to accessing health services, such as fear of disclosure, lack of trust, and denial of care. Stigma can also create barriers to adhering to health recommendations, such as reluctance to wear masks, practice social distancing, and isolate when sick.

Stigma can also create barriers to participating in research and innovation, such as refusal to enroll in clinical trials, provide samples, or share data. Stigma can also create barriers to engaging in health promotion and education, such as resistance to listen to health messages, seek information, or change behavior. Stigma can also create barriers to collaborating and cooperating with health authorities, such as distrust, hostility, and violence.

The new name "mpox" aims to promote public health by encouraging people to seek testing and vaccination, and to follow health guidelines and advice. The new name also aims to promote public health by increasing the awareness and understanding of the disease and how to prevent and control it. The new name also aims to promote public health by enhancing the research and innovation on the disease and the vaccine, and by ensuring the quality and safety of the vaccine. The new name also aims to promote public health by improving the communication and education on the disease and the vaccine, and by using evidence-based and culturally-sensitive messages and materials. The new name also aims to promote public health by strengthening the collaboration and cooperation with health authorities, and by building trust and confidence in the health system.

Addressing the evolving understanding of the disease

As our knowledge of the disease progresses, the changing of the term highlights that the disease's origin and transmission are not related to monkeys or men having sex with monkeys, but rather to a complex and dynamic interaction of biological, environmental, and social factors. The disease is caused by a new strain of the mpox virus, which belongs to the orthopoxvirus genus, along with other viruses such as smallpox, cowpox, and vaccinia. The virus is transmitted through respiratory droplets, contact with skin lesions, or contact with contaminated objects or materials.

The virus can infect humans and animals, such as rodents, primates, and livestock. The virus can cause a range of symptoms, such as fever, headache, muscle pain, rash, and lymphadenopathy. The virus can be prevented by vaccination, and treated by antiviral drugs. The virus can be detected by laboratory tests, such as polymerase chain reaction (PCR), enzyme-linked immunosorbent assay (ELISA), and immunofluorescence assay (IFA).

The new name "mpox" aims to address the evolving understanding of the disease by reflecting the current and accurate scientific and medical information on the disease and the virus. The new name also aims to address the evolving understanding of the disease by acknowledging the uncertainty and complexity of the disease and the virus, and by being open to new discoveries and insights.

The new name also aims to address the evolving understanding of the disease by emphasizing the need for continuous and rigorous research and innovation on the disease and the virus, and by being responsive and adaptive to the changing situation and context. The new name also aims to address the evolving understanding of the disease by fostering a culture of curiosity and learning among the public and the health professionals, and by being transparent and accountable in the dissemination and communication of the knowledge and evidence.

The renaming of mpox from "monkeypox" to "mpox" is a significant and timely change that highlights the importance of avoiding stigmatizing language when referring to the disease and its affected populations. The change was made to avoid confusion and discrimination, as the original name played into "racist and stigmatizing language" that harmed the dignity and rights of the people who contracted the disease. The World Health Organization (WHO) announced the change on November 28, 2022, and the new name "mpox" was adopted following a series of consultations with global experts, including virologists, epidemiologists, linguists, ethicists, and representatives of the affected communities.

The renaming of the disease is crucial for several reasons: reducing stigma, promoting public health, and addressing the evolving understanding of the disease. However, some within stigmatized communities affected by the virus argue that while the name change is a win, it may be too little, too late. The WHO's decision to rename the disease and use both names simultaneously for one year while "monkeypox" is phased out has been criticized for causing confusion and perpetuating stigma. Despite these concerns, the renaming of mpox serves as an important step in addressing the stigma and promoting public health in the fight against the disease.

Conclusion

The 2022 mpox outbreak was a serious public health emergency that had a significant impact on society. The outbreak was characterized by the emergence of a new strain of the virus, rapid spread through human networks, and the role of air travel and animal importation in its dissemination. The outbreak affected millions of people worldwide, especially men who have sex with men, and caused thousands of deaths. The outbreak also posed a threat to global health security, as it raised the risk of bioterrorism and the re-emergence of smallpox.

The outbreak was declared a public health emergency of international concern (PHEIC) by the World Health Organization, mobilizing resources and efforts to control the spread of the disease. The outbreak triggered a global response that involved different countries, regions, and organizations, with varying levels of success and failure. The response was influenced by the distribution of vaccines, changes in public behavior, and the ease of virus transmission. The response also faced many challenges, such as inequitable access, vaccine hesitancy, and criticisms of the response.

The renaming of mpox from "monkeypox" to "mpox" highlights the importance of avoiding stigmatizing language when referring to the disease and its affected populations. The change was made to avoid confusion and discrimination, as the original name played into "racist and stigmatizing language" that harmed the dignity and rights of the people who contracted the disease. The change also reflected the evolving understanding of the disease, as it acknowledged the diversity and complexity of the disease and the virus. The change also aimed to reduce stigma, promote public health, and foster solidarity among the affected communities.

In conclusion, the 2022 mpox outbreak was a significant public health emergency that had a significant impact on society. The outbreak revealed the strengths and weaknesses of the global health system, as well as the opportunities and challenges for future response efforts. The outbreak also demonstrated the need for continuous and rigorous research and innovation on the disease and the vaccine, as well as the need for effective and ethical communication and education on the disease and the vaccine. The outbreak also underscored the importance of respecting and protecting the human rights and dignity of the people who contracted the disease, as well as the importance of addressing the stigma and discrimination that they face. The outbreak also highlighted the importance of collaboration and cooperation among different countries, regions, and organizations, as well as the importance of solidarity and support among the affected communities. The outbreak also reminded us of the fragility and resilience of human life, as well as the responsibility and compassion of human society.

References

Harrison, L. B., & Norman, F. F. (2023). Mpox in 2023: Current epidemiology and management. Current Infectious Disease Reports, 25(1), 199-209.

World Health Organization. (2023). Responding to the global mpox outbreak: Ethics issues and considerations. Policy brief.

Centers for Disease Control and Prevention. (2023). Notes from the field: Transmission of mpox to nonsexual contacts - United States, 2022. MMWR. Morbidity and Mortality Weekly Report, 72(50), 1189-1190.

Centers for Disease Control and Prevention. (2023). Epidemiology of human mpox - Worldwide, 2018-2021. MMWR. Morbidity and Mortality Weekly Report, 72(3), 49-52.

Cohen, D., Levy, Y., Shemer-Avni, Y., & Mor, O. (2023). Detection of mpox virus using microbial cell-free DNA: The potential of metagenomic next-generation sequencing for emerging infectious diseases. The Journal of Infectious Diseases. Advance online publication.

www.ingramcontent.com/pod-product-compliance
Lightning Source LLC
Chambersburg PA
CBHW062249290526
45794CB00006B/2478